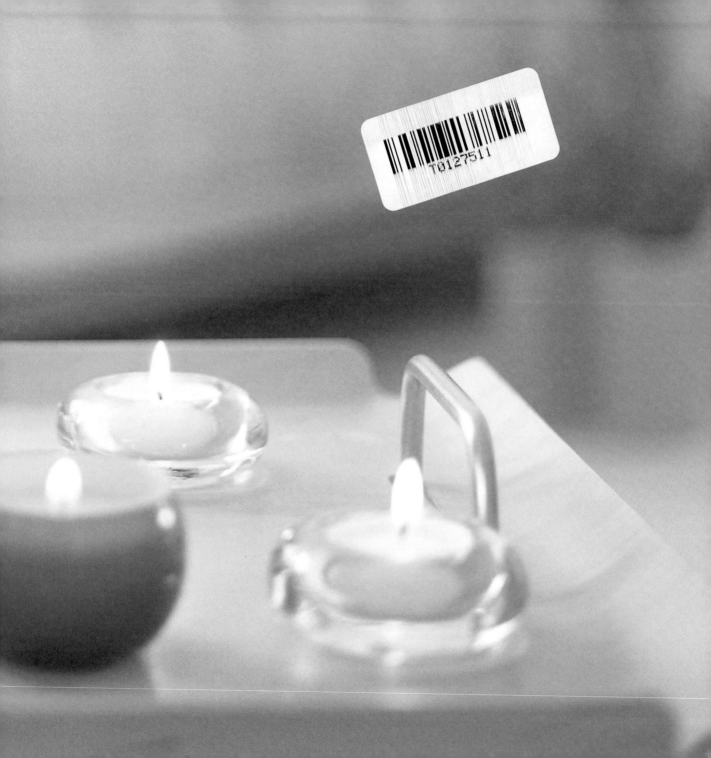

tantric sex

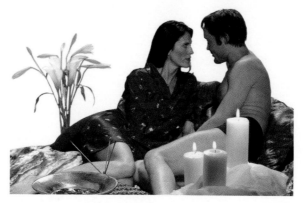

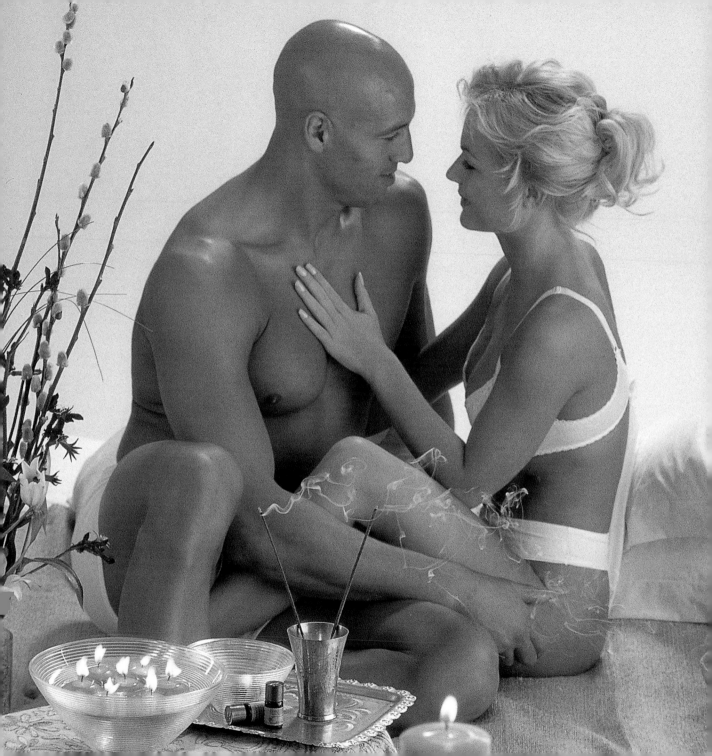

tantric sex

the ancient art of tantra
for sensual exploration

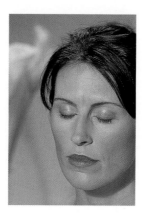

nitya lacroix

LORENZ BOOKS

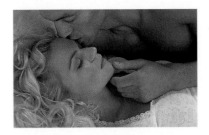

This edition is published by Lorenz Books, an imprint of Anness Publishing Ltd,
Blaby Road, Wigston, Leicestershire LE18 4SE; info@anness.com

www.lorenzbooks.com; www.annesspublishing.com

If you like the images in this book and would like to investigate using them for publishing, promotions or
advertising, please visit our website www.practicalpictures.com for more information.

Publisher: Joanna Lorenz
Editor: Debra Mayhew
Designed by: DW Design
Stylist: Claire Louise Hunt
Hair and Make-up: Nadia V. Persaud
Models: Ralph Beck, Daz Crawford, Kay Marshall, Kerry Anne Martin
Production Controller: Steve Lang
Main photography by: Alistair Hughes
Additional photos by: Michelle Garrett

© Anness Publishing Limited 2013

SAFER-SEX PRACTICES
It is wise for all sexual partners to follow the medical guidelines of safer sex practices to protect themselves from
sexually transmitted diseases, including the HIV virus which can develop into AIDS. Always avoid the exchange
of body fluids, which include vaginal secretions, semen and blood, by using latex condoms and a spermicide.

PUBLISHER'S NOTE
Although the advice and information in this book are believed to be accurate and true at the time of going to
press, neither the authors nor the publisher can accept any legal responsibility or liability for any errors or
omissions that may have been made nor for any inaccuracies nor for any loss, harm or injury that comes about
from following instructions or advice in this book.

CONTENTS

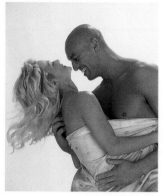

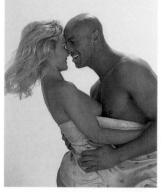

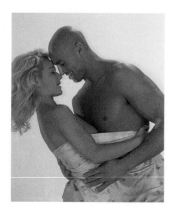

INTRODUCTION

To follow the path of tantric loving is to take a holistic approach to your partnership. By dedicating yourselves mind, body and spirit to your relationship, you are making a mutual commitment to enhance its happiness and intimacy. The modern tantric path derives its influences from the ancient Eastern tradition of Tantra, but many of its concepts remain relevant for the modern couple. Indeed, with all the stresses that impinge on our lives today, couples often need to find imaginative ways to preserve and

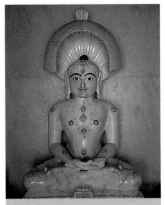

▲ *This statue depicts the pathway of the energy centres in the body.*

develop the equilibrium within their relationships. Tantric loving helps you to create a safe haven within your hearts and the privacy of your home to foster a deep sense of respect and love for each other.

Tantric loving is not simply a sexual technique, but rather a commitment to live a more conscious life in every respect. It has a spiritual dimension, even though it does not require a specific belief or religious viewpoint. It perceives a sexual relationship to be not only the physical union of two people, but

▼ *Emotional and physical harmony is enhanced by a meditative and tantric approach to love-making.*

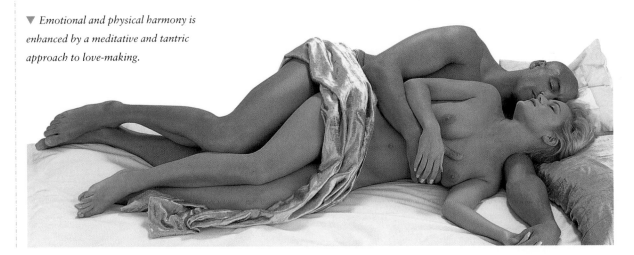

a re-enactment of the divine principle of union that governs the whole of Existence. Tantra teaches that it is the perfect merging of the cosmic male principle with the cosmic female principle that creates universal harmony and equilibrium. So tantric love-making is an invitation to the sacred mystery of the universe to enter into sexual intercourse.

This book does not aim to reveal or teach the disciplines and secrets of traditional Tantra, which began to flourish in parts of India and Tibet about 5,000 years ago. True disciples would spend years under the guidance of a teacher to initiate them into the progressive series of esoteric practices, known as "Kundalini-yoga". These practices include advanced yogic postures and breathing techniques, meditation, chanting and sexual yoga for the purpose of attaining a state of spiritual enlightenment or cosmic consciousness. This book's purpose is to take and adapt some of

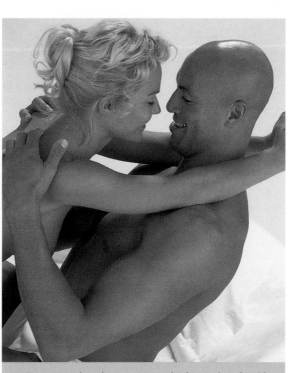

▲ *Tantra teaches that your sexual relationship should be filled with pleasure and joy. Relax and have fun and always bring laughter and playfulness into your sexual interaction.*

the basic concepts of tantric loving that may help to enhance the ecstasy of your love-making.

There is a temperance in the passion of tantric love-making which makes it qualitatively different from normal sexual activity. To experience this alternative way of making love may require you to change your established patterns of sexual behaviour, but remember that the teachings of Tantra do not exclude or make judgement on any kind of sexual activity as long as it is embarked upon in the spirit of love and mutual pleasure. Tantra perceives that all sexual relationships contain the essential element of merging and union, and therefore have the potential for a higher spiritual experience. Explore tantric love-making at a pace that suits you both. Do not put pressure on each other to achieve any kind of pre-set goal, and do not deny yourselves the type of sexual activity you have always enjoyed. Ritualize your tantric love-making in the ways described so that you do not confuse it with the occasions when you want to indulge in excitement and hot passion, fast sex, fantasy sex and the quick orgasm. As you increasingly allow stillness and meditation into your love-making your sexual ecstacy will start to become more profound. Most of all, remember that the love life you forge with your beloved is unique to your own relationship. Let that relationship be full of joy and playfulness as you embark on the sensual adventure of tantric loving.

A major emphasis in tantric love-making is on the man's retention of his orgasm. In some schools of traditional Eastern thought, the man is advised to

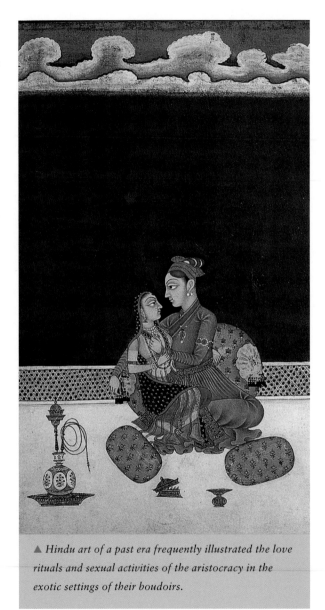

▲ Hindu art of a past era frequently illustrated the love rituals and sexual activities of the aristocracy in the exotic settings of their boudoirs.

withhold his ejaculation completely, releasing it not more than three times in ten sexual episodes. According to tantric, and Chinese Taoist teachings, the ejaculation of semen causes a depletion of vital life energy which weakens the man, both spiritually and physically. Tantra, in particular, teaches that the energy of orgasm can be harnessed as a force for inner trans-formation. Instead of dissipating semen the man should moderate his excitement, and through the use of breath and thought control draw the force of his orgasmic energy upwards so that it ascends towards the brain, opening up internal psychic energy centres to bring him to a higher state of realization.

▶ *The erotic sculptures of the Konarak and Khajuraho temples in India depict the ascent of the human spirit from ordinary copulation to a transcendental state of sexual union.*

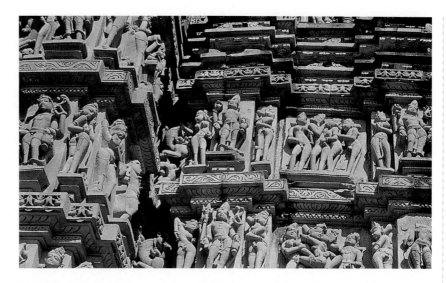

▼ *In tantric love-making, the man surrenders himself into the energy of the woman, adoring her with every touch, without losing control of his passions.*

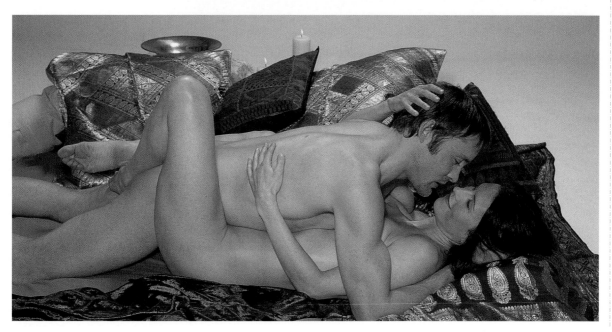

THE CHAKRAS

The concept of a subtle energy body is an important principle in Tantra. For centuries, Eastern philosophies, religions and healing traditions have recognized that an etheric energy body exists parallel to the physical body. There are seven major energy centres, known as chakras, located in specific areas of this energy body. These chakras interact with the existential universal forces, which are governed by a divine Cosmic Consciousness. The human body, then, according to Tantra, is a hallowed temple that contains the energetic potential to merge with a state of cosmic bliss. Conscious sexuality, says Tantra, unleashes a powerful force within the body, known as "Kundalini energy". The Kundalini is active female creative energy manifested in all universal matter. Normally, the Kundalini lies dormant within us, but when it is awakened by yogic practices, meditation and sexual activity, it ascends through the energy body on its potential journey to the crown chakra, the seat of cosmic oneness and bliss. Each chakra is associated with one of the rainbow colours, see right, and with a certain level of vibration.

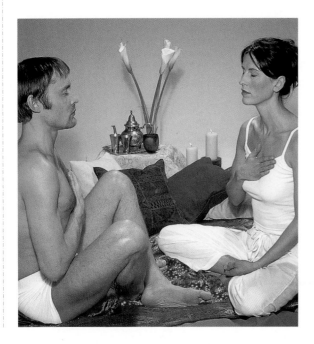

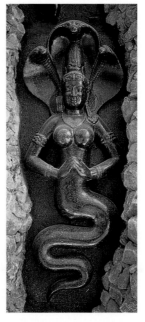

◀ *The Kundalini sexual energy in Tantra is a feminine creative force often portrayed as an uncoiled serpent.*

◀ FAR LEFT: *Sit together and breathe meditatively into each chakra. Focus especially on the heart chakra, which is the energy centre for love, merging and empathy.*

Located between the eyebrows, Ajna is often referred to as the "third eye" and is the seat of intuition or "sixth sense". It is associated with higher knowledge, intellect and compassion. Indigo.

Located above the crown of the head, Sahasrara is associated with self-realization, cosmic consciousness, bliss and total unity with the whole. Violet.

Located between the nipples, the heart chakra or Anahat relates to love, empathy, joy and the union of body and spirit, as well as the merging of male and female polar energies. Green.

Located in the throat, Vishuddha is associated with self-awareness, purity, expression and communication. Blue.

Located just below the navel, Swadhishtana is the source of vital life energy, and is the core centre of balance and gravity within us. It relates to emotion, reproduction and sexual drive. Orange.

The Manipur or solar plexus chakra resides at a central point beneath the rib cage and is associated with intellect, power, will, ego and action. Yellow.

Located at the base of the sex organs, the base chakra or Muladhara is associated with survival and sexuality, pain and pleasure. Red.

EQUILIBRIUM AND HARMONY

The search for union and harmony is at the heart of tantric teaching. It seeks to restore equilibrium between the polar masculine and feminine forces which govern the whole of Existence. According to Tantra, the relationship between a man and woman is a microcosmic enactment of the fundamental law which rules the whole of the Universe. Strife occurs when these two opposing energies are discordant with each other. When they are in harmony, the polar energies complement each other and merge as one. Bliss, says Tantra, arises out of the state of perfect union.

A tantric relationship is one that enjoys a deep emotional and sexual intimacy and is built on a strong foundation of honest and sincere communication. Mutual trust is essential if openness, confidence and respect – all fundamental ingredients of an intimately bonded partnership – are to flourish.

These qualities are not necessarily present in the first flush of sexual excitement that invariably accompanies the beginnings of a relationship. Passion can easily override other considerations and, while it has a vitality and binding energy of its own, its very nature is one of transience. Holistic loving is more enduring and is rooted in the acceptance of our own and the other person's humanity. We all have our own particular strengths and weaknesses, and respecting and caring for these qualities in another person establishes the basis of equality in a relationship so that the games of power and manipulation cannot take hold.

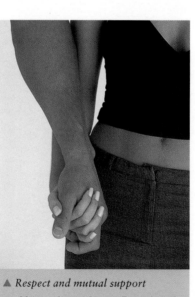

▲ *Respect and mutual support enables a relationship to flourish and mature in ways that benefit and bring strength to both sexes.*

Intimacy develops when we share our thoughts, feelings and bodies with our beloved. We cannot hide away one part of ourselves and expect to be available and open with another. Lovers should reach out to each other in a holistic way, bringing heart, mind, body and soul into their communion. Sometimes this is painful because we may have to lower the defences we have carefully constructed against the hurts and bruises of life, and perhaps experienced in previous relationships. It may require deep and honest soul-searching to find within ourselves the causes of our own internal pain, so that we do not always blame the other person for our difficulties or neediness. It takes tolerance and generosity of imagination to understand that the other person's needs and opinions may be different from our own. It demands courage to speak honestly and clearly about what we are feeling and what we personally need from the relationship. The organic growth of intimacy must be constantly

nurtured. We cannot afford to fix our loved one or ourselves into a comfortable rut, for each of us has our own personal destiny as well as the destiny we share with each other. Our emotional and sexual lives are undoubtedly enriched when we are able to reveal the truth of who we are, and in doing so find a deep and genuine acceptance of each other.

▼ *The capacity to be vulnerable with each other enables great tenderness to develop between you.*

▼ *Let your combined masculine and feminine strengths become a complementary influence in your relationship.*

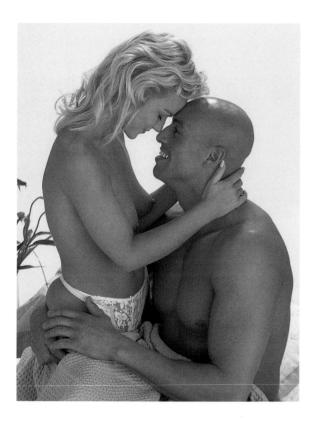

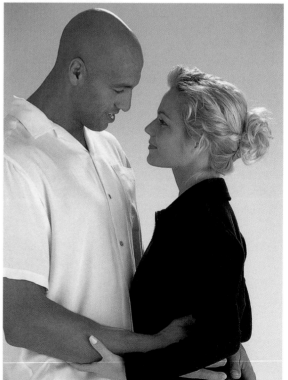

EMOTIONAL HONESTY

Resolving issues of conflict as and when they arise between yourself and your partner will ensure that your love-making stays spontaneous and unimpeded by hidden resentments and anger which might otherwise create tensions between you. Tantric loving is an holistic experience. You cannot give yourself wholeheartedly to the sexual experience if you are holding back on an emotional level. Committing yourselves to setting aside quality time for discussing underlying problems and comprehending each other's point of view will help all aspects of your relationship to remain healthy. Communicating and listening to each other in a positive way, in spite of the difficult issues that need to be discussed, is a relationship skill. It does not always come easily and you may need to suspend rigid opinions in order to hear and respond to the feelings of your partner.

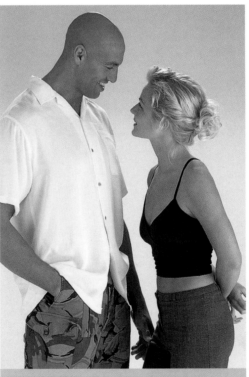

▲ *The willingness to communicate your feelings instils vitality into your relationship.*

When you feel that the need is there, allocate a period of time to discuss the issues that are troubling you and causing conflict. Each partner should have a precise period (between 5-10 minutes at any one time) to discuss their issues calmly and without interruption. The other partner should listen carefully to what is being said, trying to remain receptive to the other's words without becoming defensive. When it is your turn, you will have the opportunity to put forward your own point of view in the secure knowledge that you, too, will be heard calmly and without interruption. Be conscious of your body language, adopting a posture that is relaxed and open so that your stance is not intimidating, closed or submissive, but instead welcomes communication and an exchange of views.

▶ *Talk clearly and simply about what you need and want. Take responsibility by placing your words in the context of "I" rather than "you". Accusation and blame will only alienate him.*

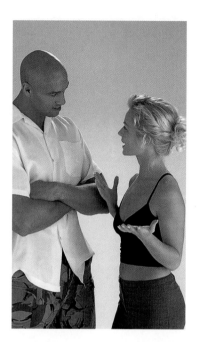

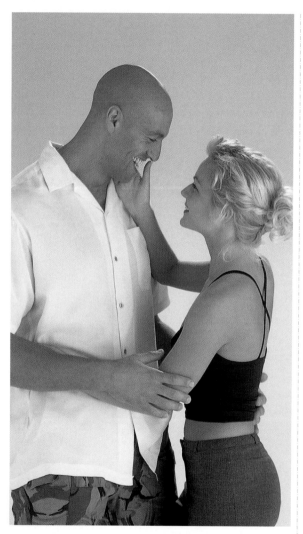

▶ *When talking, try not to dominate by raising your voice or being condescending. Do not be afraid to show your vulnerability. Trust that she will listen to you.*

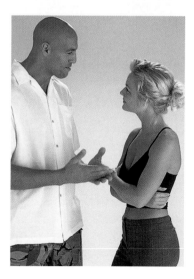

▲ *Indicate through body language that you are supportive. Leaning towards your partner, maintaining eye contact and taking his or her hand in your own are gestures that show that you are interested in their point of view.*

THE JOY OF SEXUAL SHARING

Your sexuality is a precious and intrinsic part of your nature, and deserves to be treated with respect. In an intimate and tantric relationship, lovers should be able to trust each other implicitly with their bodies and their sexuality. When mutual reverence is there, there are no sexual boundaries or rules except for those decided upon by the two individuals concerned.

Physical intimacy develops as you open up to each other, sharing your sexual thoughts, feelings, fears, desires and fantasies. Create time to talk to one another about these things, but do so only when there is no underlying tension between you. Never criticize

each other sexually, or use sexual secrets shared between you against each other.

Find ways to show each other what you like and want sexually in an atmosphere of playfulness and co-operation. Go to the bedroom together, not specifically to have sexual intercourse, but to explore new realms of physical pleasure and to discover more about each other's sexual preferences.

▼ *Exploring every inch of his skin with your lips will increase his sensual awareness of his body and enlighten you to his sexual responses.*

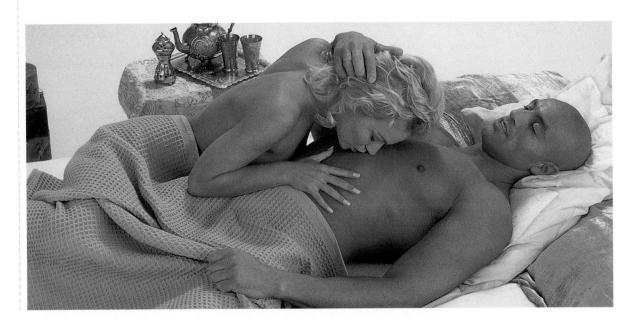

Choose a time when there are no outside pressures or interruptions, and when neither of you is tired.

Touch and stroke each other, using different means of tactile contact such as your lips, tongue, fingers and body parts, so that you become familiar with all of your partner's body. Tell each other in what manner and where you especially like to be touched and kissed. Show each other how you want to be caressed and stimulated on your most intimate areas. Guide each other on how to stroke, lick and kiss the genital parts to increase arousal. Male and female sexual needs and responses can vary greatly, so learn from each other the different ways to bring sexual joy to a partner of the opposite sex.

▼ *Learn from her how and where she loves to be touched and caressed by you, and take pleasure in her whole body erogeny.*

Play-act some of your erotic fantasies together. Be open to experimenting with something new, but always be respectful of your own or your partner's boundaries. Never pressurize your lover into performing a sexual act against his or her will. Sharing these sexual intimacies, and revealing yourselves in this way, enables you both to relax deeply with each other. While fantasy and excitement is not the essence of tantric love-making, you should first be able to embrace and enjoy all aspects of your sexuality without guilt or judgement. Always treasure the information that your lover imparts about his or her sexuality. In the same way, you should honour your own sexual uniqueness.

▼ *Sexual tension dissolves more easily if you are able to be playful with each other on a physical level.*

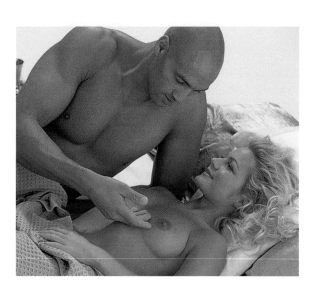

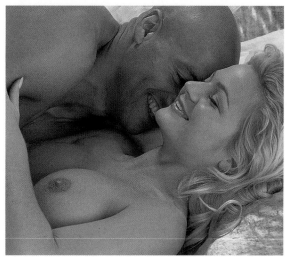

THE ART OF AROUSAL

Sexual wisdom acknowledges that a man's passion is generally aroused more quickly than a woman's and is faster to reach its climax, while a woman's sexual arousal is slower to ignite but endures longer. In the art of love-making, the couple should aim to harmonize these differences so that the progress of their sexual arousal becomes more balanced, and enables them to reach mutual satisfaction. In tantric love-making, great emphasis is placed on a woman's natural right to reach her peak of sexual ecstasy. The man must therefore learn to pace his passion and to make love to his partner selflessly and, by doing so, his patience is rewarded by his partner's joy.

The art of arousal is in the sensual awakening of the body as a whole, and in the presence of being that you bring into your every touch and caress. Experience each moment of physical contact for its own pleasurable sake rather than as a means to an end. Do not rush into intercourse or hurry towards your climax, but rather lose yourselves in the joy of extended sensual foreplay. Take time to hold each other and breathe slowly and deeply together, establishing eye contact on occasions to strengthen your intimacy and emotional connection. When you do close your eyes, concentrate on the sensations that each kiss and caress stirs within you and savour the pleasure of each one.

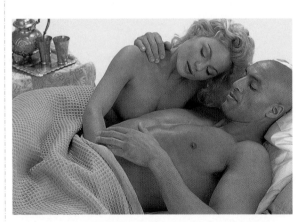

▲ *Not every touch has to excite. Arousal levels can be allowed to rise and fall naturally. Linger enjoyably by tenderly and teasingly stroking intimate parts of his body.*

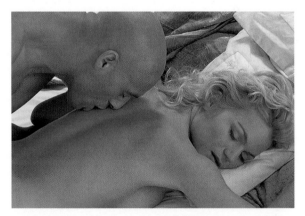

▲ *She will love to feel your kisses covering every inch of her skin. Let your lips brush and anoint the back of her body, and tease her intimate areas.*

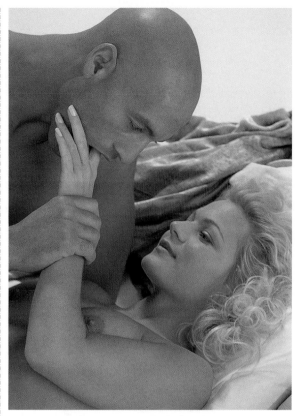

▲ *Every part of her body is worthy of your attention and is erotically sensitive. Take her fingertips into your mouth one by one; suck them gently, rolling your tongue around them.*

▶ *Kiss as if engaged in the act of making love itself. The mouth, lips and tongue are highly erotically charged, and when they meet with willingness and receptivity there is a fusion of your male and female sexual energies.*

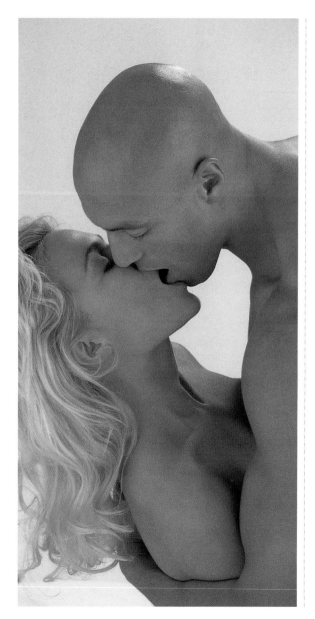

FEMALE EROTICISM

When a man makes love to a woman, he should do so in a manner of reverence and adoration, perceiving her body as both a temple of delight and an altar of devotion. Tantric texts describe a woman's sexuality as a sacred mystery and a medium through which both she and her male partner can attain physical and spiritual ecstasy.

A woman's whole body is erotogenic and she is especially sensitive to touch, so her lover should bestow his kisses and caresses on every part of her. Her sexuality is awakened by and responsive to not only his physical embraces, but also to her sense of being emotionally cherished. A sensitive lover ensures that the woman is fully sexually aroused through loving, mutual foreplay before he enters her. In a state of arousal, a woman's nipples may become erect, her skin may flush and her vaginal juices will start to flow. Through her words, her sighs and her body's responses, she signals to her lover that she is emotionally and physically ready to receive him.

In historic Eastern manuscripts relating to sexuality, many elaborate terms were employed to describe a woman's most intimate sexual organs — the vagina and clitoris. Names such as Jewel or Lotus (a sacred Indian flower) are found in the Hindu Tantra, while the Chinese Taoist tradition used poetic terms such as the Jade Gate, the Valley of Joy and Pearl. These elaborate names illustrate the respect accorded to a woman's erotic nature and show that her sexual organs were perceived as the divine gateway to joy.

◀ *Her whole body will long for your caresses so embrace all parts of her, not just certain specific erogenous zones. Stroke and squeeze her legs and feet as they will be sensitve to your touch.*

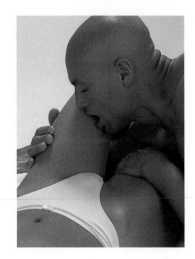

◀ *The areas which surround her sexual organs are also erotically charged. Honour this part of her with kisses and sensual touches which anoint her thighs and belly.*

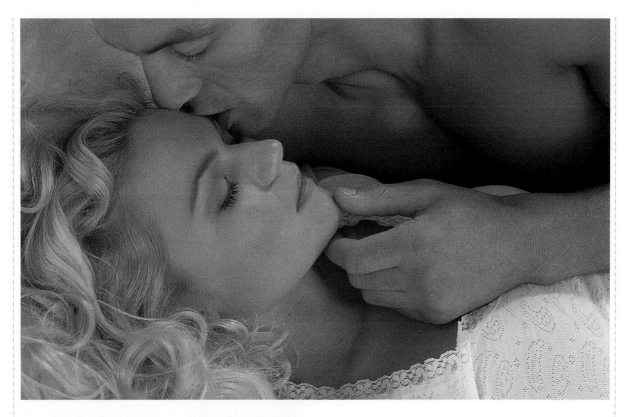

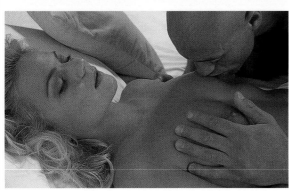

▲ *Tenderly plant your kisses on to her face, letting them brush her forehead, ears and eyes before your lips meet. These intimate gestures will open her heart to you.*

◄ *Her breasts are highly erogenous and as you kiss and lick them, and suck her nipples, you will arouse her sexually. Always touch her breasts with respect.*

MALE EROTICISM

Visual stimulus generally plays a considerable part in male sexual arousal, as does direct tactile contact to the man's major erogenous area – the penis. Without direct stimulation to the penis and its sensitive tip, the glans, it is difficult for a man to reach an orgasm. It is an essential part of the art of love-making that his lover understands how to move her pelvis during intercourse, or to kiss and caress his sexual organ, so that he gains maximum pleasure without coming to a premature climax. She should seek to learn from her partner what manner of erotic strokes and movements bring him sexual happiness, and to learn from his signals when to slow the pace.

Culture has tended to deny men the same opportunity of experiencing whole body sensuality that it has allowed women to enjoy. From an early age, men are often conditioned into being hardened and detached from the body, except in the realm of competition, stamina and physical prowess. The more subtle nuances of physical and tactile sensuality, which are so much a part of sensitive tantric love-making, are often neglected. In ancient tantric rituals, it was customary for the male disciple to bathe and anoint his body before participating in sexual ceremonies. He would engage in elaborate rites, touching specific parts of his body while chanting significant sounds intended to heighten his physical, spiritual and energetic responses to his sexual partner.

▲ *Do not focus your attention too directly towards his genital organs. First tease and stimulate him, nuzzling, licking and kissing his belly and thighs to arouse this erotically charged area.*

A man who wishes to embark on the journey of holistic love-making will need to become more physically sensual and sensitive to his own body. He should also enjoy the erotic whole-body contact of extended foreplay for its own sake, surrendering to his lover's kisses and strokes so that his sexual consciousness floods through every part of him.

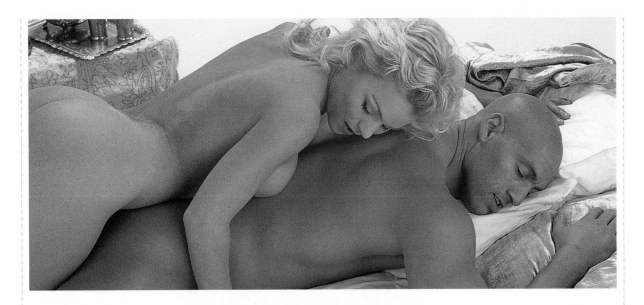

▲ *He will love this playful yet totally sexy feeling of your body writhing over his skin. It will make him aware of the sensuality of the back of his body as your breasts and belly roll over him.*

▶ *Stimulate him on and around his buttocks. Caressing and kneading these fleshy muscles can be sexually arousing for him, as is stroking his perineum and scrotum.*

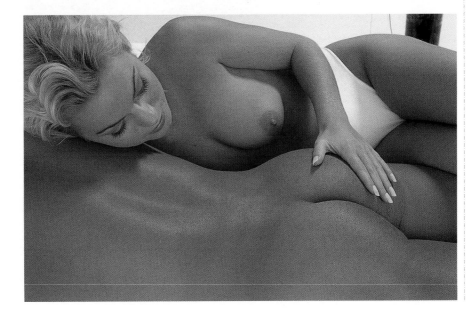

23

RITUALS OF DEVOTION

Tantric loving is full of little ritual acts of devotion because this is one way to keep alive the respect and love in a partnership, and so continue to honour each other. In traditional Tantra, the initiates would offer one another gifts of flowers, food and wine before taking part in sexual ceremonies. They would also anoint each other, and massage and touch each other's bodies. These rites were performed because, to the tantric disciple, the lover personified a divine presence.

The elaborate forms of ritual helped focus the minds of the disciples on the sacredness of sexuality. Tantric sex is all about conscious love-making. Sexual partners must prepare themselves and their environment with the full awareness that they are to engage in a physical act that is essentially spiritual in content.

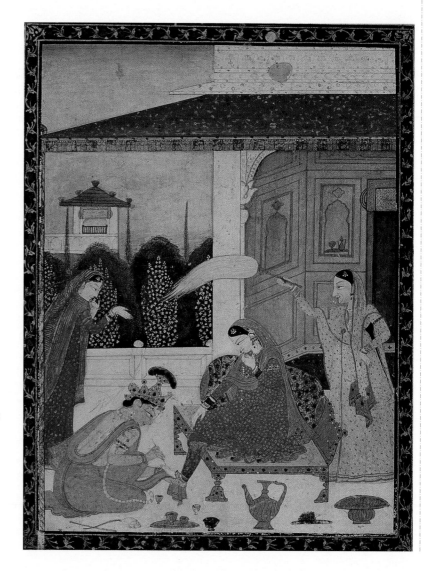

▶ *Hindu art shows the allure of a devoted lover honouring his goddess.*

PERFUMES OF LOVE

Tantric lovers have always used fragrance in their ceremonial rituals. According to tantric teachings, smell is the sense that ignites sexual energy. In traditional tantric sexual ceremonies, fragrant potions blended from woods, plants and herbs were used to anoint the bodies of lovers and to heighten both physical sensuality and spiritual awareness. Today you can create your own perfumes of love from the wide selection of aromatic essential oils available in pharmacies and health shops. Once you understand their effects and properties you can use them to enhance your sexual relationship.

Essential oils are essences distilled from a variety of natural resources such as flowers, herbs, fruits, leaves, roots, sap and the bark of trees. The essences contain many of the healing properties of their source plants, and their specific aromas can transform the mood of lovers and create an atmosphere conducive to transcendental love-making. Sandalwood and camphor are two of the most popular ceremonial fragrances, while frankincense and cedarwood have always been associated with religious significance and worship. Jasmine and rose have long been associated with love and seduction.

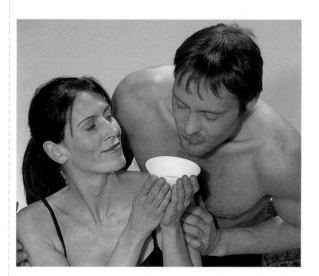

▲ *Select the aromatic oils which most appeal to you and your lover's sense of smell and mood.*

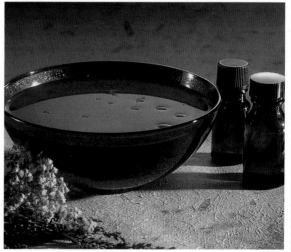

▲ *When you prepare to give a massage, add a few drops of fragranced essential oils into the basic carrier.*

AROMATICS FOR INTIMACY

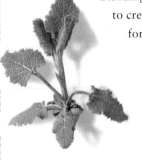

▲ *Clary sage*

Blending aromatic essences in order to create a fragrant atmosphere for love, and to enhance sensuality, introduces the important aspect of ritual into your love-making. Aromatic essences, blended to evoke positive changes in body, mind and soul, contribute to that intention.

Develop a sound knowledge of the effects of each fragrance, and of the physical and mental benefits of the essences' properties. Be guided by your instinctive response to the individual aromas and their combined smells. Soon you will notice how certain fragrances influence mood, instil calm, stimulate the physical senses, arouse sexual feeling or create a meditative atmosphere. Those recipes that work on you and your lover holistically are the ones that

▲ *Ginger* are most compatible to tantric love-making. Use no more than three essential oils together at any one time or your sense of smell will become overwhelmed.

Certain aromatic essences have a long-established reputation for their aphrodisiac qualities: SANDALWOOD has a woody, sweet fragrance that has a sensual effect on the body and a calming influence on the mind. Like sandalwood, patchouli originates from India and was used traditionally in tantric ritual. Its enduring musky smell is relaxing yet sexually evocative. JASMINE, which opens its heavenly scented flowers at night, has long been associated with the powerful influences of love.

▼ *Sandalwood*

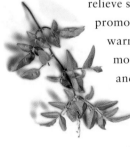

Jasmine absolute has particularly good effects on male sexuality, helping to relieve sexual tensions and to promote physical and emotional warmth. ROSE ABSOLUTE is the most feminine of fragrances and is associated with love, healing and seduction. It weaves its sweet magic to dissolve emotional wounds and

▲ *Jasmine* encourage the heart to trust

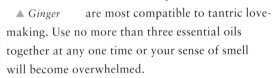

again. The haunting, bittersweet perfume of NEROLI ABSOLUTE, drawn from orange blossom, is said to soothe sexual anxieties while boosting virility and fertility. It blends beautifully with rose and jasmine to make a seductive aromatic recipe for love-making. YLANG-YLANG exudes a sweet, exotic fragrance and deserves its erotic reputation; only a few drops should be used as its heady scent can be quite overpowering. BASIL, which also originates from India, is a restorative essential oil with a reputation for igniting sexual energy. BENZOIN, BLACK PEPPER and GINGER bring warmth to the heart and body, and CLARY SAGE adds a touch of euphoria.

▲ *Juniper*

▲ *Benzoin*

▼ *Lavender*

Citrus-derived essences such as LIME, ORANGE and BERGAMOT add zest and an aspect of playfulness to your love life.

Some aromatic essences, such as LAVENDER and GERANIUM, are not in themselves aphrodisiacs but instead enhance the mood of equilibrium that is so vital for harmonious love-making. JUNIPER is soothing and helps to relieve anxiety and nervous tension. The resinous scent of FRANKINCENSE and the woody aroma of CEDARWOOD both instil calm and serenity, and so are conducive to elevating the mind and enhancing the spiritual focus of your sexual activity. Indeed, cedar is a Semitic word which means "the power of spiritual strength".

Always select good-quality essential oils, storing them in a cool place and away from sunlight. Keep blended oils in darkened glass bottles or porcelain containers, but not in a plastic container as they may react against its chemical composition. Never apply essential oils directly on to the skin, but dilute according to prescription with a natural vegetable oil such as grapeseed, sunflower or almond. Aromatic essences are potent substances and should be used according to the instructions of the manufacturers or the advice of a qualified aromatherapist. Seek advice on the use and contra-indications of essential oils if you are pregnant, sick, frail or elderly, or prone to skin sensitivity.

SENSUAL AROMATICS

Essential oils can be used in a variety of ways to cast their gentle spell on your love life. Before making love, bathe alone or together with your partner in water infused with up to seven drops of aphrodisiac and relaxing essential oils. Blend the drops into a teaspoon of almond oil and add the mixture to the water once the bath has filled. Stir the water thoroughly so the essences are well dispersed then relax into it, breathing deeply to inhale the aromas. Select essences that are kind to the skin and that you are sure will not cause a skin allergy.

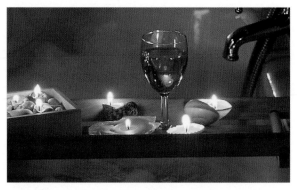

▲ *Combining candles and fragrance in the bathroom intoxicates the senses.*

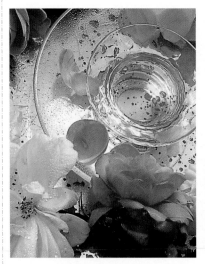

▲ *The perfume of essential oil and flowers instils romance.*

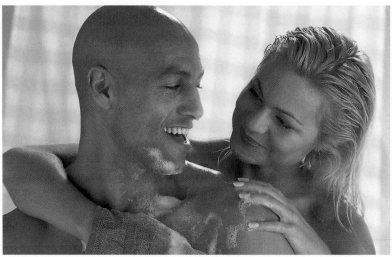

▲ *Aromatic soaps and lotions make bathing a sensual experience.*

By using an aroma burner, you can infuse your special love chamber with a subtle and inviting fragrance. Add your selected blend of seven essential oil drops to the bowl of water and light the tea-candle beneath it so that the enticing scented vapour impregnates the atmosphere. Aromatherapy candles can also be used for the same purpose.

Aromatic essences can be added to a pure vegetable oil to deepen the tender experience of a loving whole-body massage, which you can give to or receive from your partner. Massage between lovers can be an experience of emotional and physical relaxation, or enjoyed as a prelude to love-making. Create a romantic, uplifting and sensually inspiring recipe of essential oils, mixing between 12-14 drops of essences into 25 ml/1 fl oz/1$^1/_2$ tsp of vegetable oil.

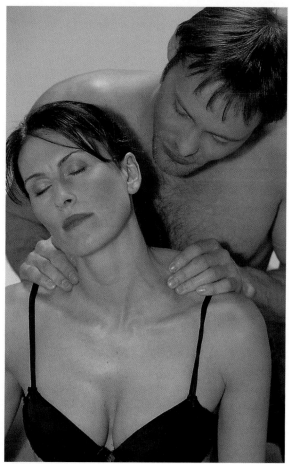

▲ *The combined effects of massage strokes and the aromatic influence of scented oils will dispel her tension and help her to relax.*

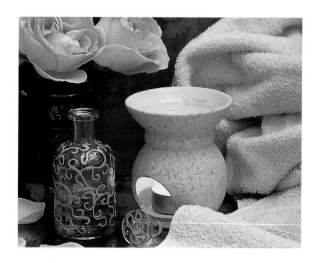

◄ *A lighted aroma burner will infuse the room with fragrance, but do be careful not to leave the lighted candle unattended.*

THE TOUCH OF LOVE

Touch is one of the most profound means of communication between two people. The laying of loving hands upon the body conveys a depth of feeling that goes way beyond the impact of words. Touch has a direct link with your inner world of feelings, and through it you can express your affection, your concern, your pleasure and appreciation. To receive the benefits of caring touch upon your body is also a deeply moving experience. The power of nurturing touch imparts the healing effects of wholeness and integration, and thus restores a sense of balance and equilibrium between body, mind and spirit.

Explore the world of touch in ways that are not solely confined to an act of sexual arousal. Touching each other with respect, with tenderness, with sensuality and with playfulness will greatly strengthen your physical and emotional intimacy. Learn some of the basic strokes of massage so that you become confident and skilled in the art of touch. Through massage, your hands can relax your lover's body, easing away its tensions and restoring a sense of mental peace. Massage revitalizes the whole physical system, awakens sensuality and enlivens the skin to its full capacity of feeling. It is the perfect gift for partners to bestow upon each other.

Prepare a relaxing and welcoming environment in which to give a massage. Ensure that the room is warm and well ventilated, and that the lighting is soft and soothing. A mattress or duvet placed on the floor

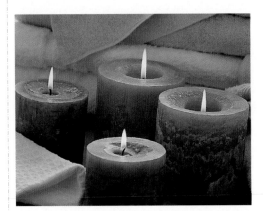

▲ *The soft glow of candles will create a soothing atmosphere in which to massage your beloved.*

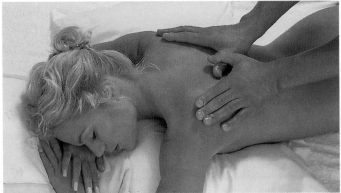

▲ *Massage is a gift to share, and can be used to soothe and relax, while enhancing your emotional and physical bond.*

will provide greater support and freedom of movement than massaging on the bed. Cover the base with freshly laundered sheets or bath towels to protect it from excess oil, and keep clean towels and

▼ *Your partner will appreciate the special care that you have taken in preparing a welcoming massage environment.*

a blanket close by to cover your partner if necessary.

Use your essential oils to create a fragrant ambience. Add your chosen blend either to an aroma burner to infuse the atmosphere, or to the massage oil. Music will enhance the mood of relaxation and romance, but ensure your choice of music does not impose on the calming effects of your strokes.

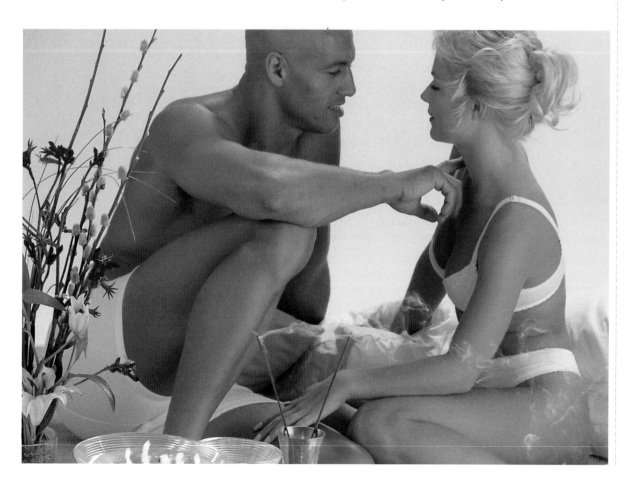

TENDER STROKES

The most important element of massage is the caring quality of presence and feeling that you bring to your hands as you touch your lover's body. Trust your hands and follow your sense of intuition which will show you how and where to apply your strokes. You will gain confidence if you learn some of the basic techniques from books or a massage class, but the essence of healing comes from deep within you when your feelings of love and tenderness flow through your hands without any inhibition. Your touch can be firm yet gentle, nurturing yet playful, sensual yet comforting. Always massage your lover with respect, honouring their body as it rests before you. This is the way to make your massage a truly tantric experience.

Take care of your own body while giving a massage. Be alert to your own comfort, ensuring that your posture remains aligned, open and relaxed, and that your breathing is deep and easy. If you feel peaceful and relaxed within yourself, your massage will have a meditative quality that will benefit you both. Apply your strokes in a rhythmic and fluid manner, emphasizing the roundness and sensuality of your lover's body, and moving your hands from one area to another so that they convey a sense of whole-body integration. Let your hands be soft and supple, even when applying a stronger pressure, and imagine that they are sculpting your lover's body rather than imposing upon it.

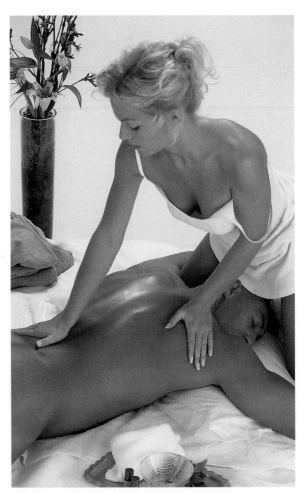

1 *Spread the oil smoothly with flowing strokes over the area of the body you are about to massage. Use this time to relax and become attuned to each other.*

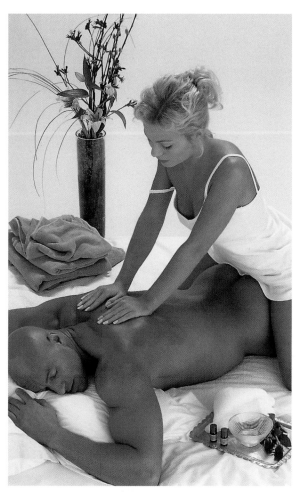

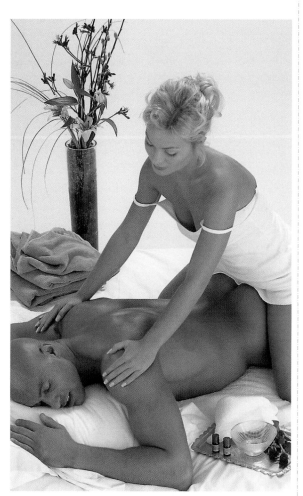

2 *A long, sweeping stroke over the back can be performed while straddling the hips of your partner. This ensures close contact, but take care to support your own weight.*

3 *Your massage can be both therapeutic and sensual. Your hands should always encompass fully the contours of the body, such as the shoulders, hips and buttocks.*

SENSUAL STROKES

Some of the most sensual massage strokes can be repeated over many different parts of the body, adapting them to the size of the area and varying their pace and pressure. In this way, you are able to build up a repertoire of soothing and sensual motions from relatively few simple strokes. The gentle strokes shown here create a hypnotic and relaxing effect, enabling your partner to surrender fully to the caress of your loving hands. In addition, they prepare, warm and enliven the body so that it becomes more responsive to touch. Repeat each sequence of strokes three times before gliding smoothly into the next movement.

FAN STROKES

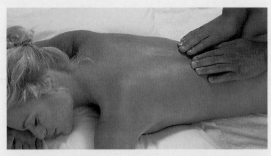

1 To fan stroke up the back, rest both palms flat on each side of the spine. Steadily slide your hands upwards for a distance of about 15 cm (6 in).

FEATHERING

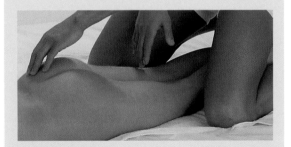

Feather touches produce a pleasurable, teasing sensation on the skin. Stroke your fingertips lightly downwards, one hand overlapping the other, to stimulate the skin's sensory nerves.

CIRCLE STROKES

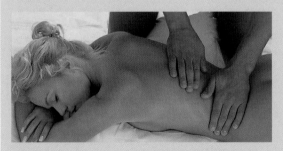

1 Place both hands parallel but slightly apart, fingers pointing away from you, on the back or belly. Slide steadily in a clockwise circular motion, right hand leading.

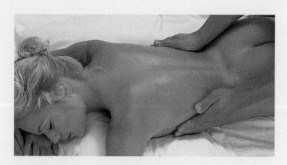

2 Fan both hands softly out towards the sides of the body so that they mould to the rib cage before pulling them firmly back downwards.

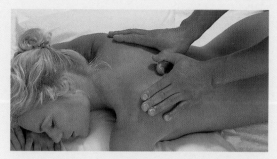

3 Flex your wrists to return your hands back to the initial position of the stroke. Glide them up to a higher level of the back and repeat the stroke.

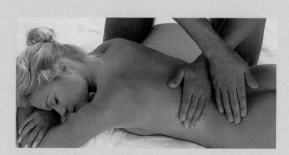

2 Lift your right hand to allow the left one to make a continuous circular motion. Pass your right hand over the left wrist before dropping it back down to complete a half-circle motion.

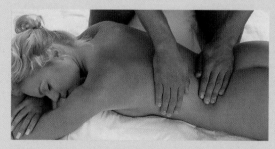

3 Continue your circle strokes so that they spiral over the surface of the skin in an unbroken motion. Remember to keep the left hand moving on the body while the right one lifts and returns.

MASSAGING INTIMATE AREAS

Massage can be a sensual prelude to love-making, especially if your hands know how to arouse the erotic areas of the body with loving strokes. It is important, however, that your touch honours your lover's body as a whole and does not overly focus on the erogenous zones. Your hands should be undemanding, tender and sensitive as you anoint the most intimate parts of the body. It is better not to over-excite your partner, but instead let your touch awaken the body's sensual responses so that the sexual energy begins to flow like a gentle stream throughout its entirety. When the massage precedes love-making, your hands should be making love to every inch of your partner's skin. From fingertips to

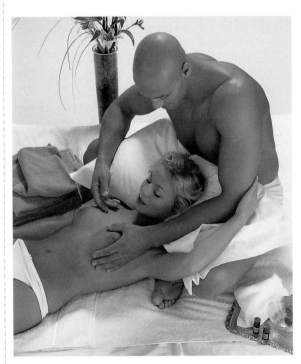

▲ *Soften your hands to gently cup and stroke over the fullness of her breasts.*

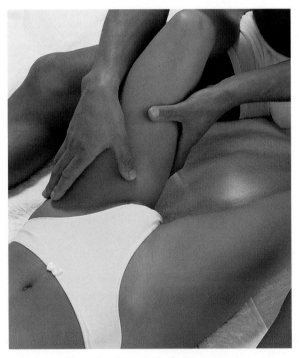

▲ *Warm and relax her thighs with the flowing motion of your strokes to ease away tension.*

toes, your touch should revere both the body and the essential being of your lover. Your strokes should never go against your lover's wishes, nor should you try to manipulate the massage towards a sexual end without your partner's willing consent. In tantric love-making there is no goal in mind except pleasure and delight in the tactile experience of the moment.

If you are the man giving the sensual massage, be gentle with your touch on your partner's breasts. Your hands can cup her breasts and your fingers can lovingly caress over her nipples, but do not linger gratuitously on this area. Instead let this erotic touch be integrated into

▶ *Stroke sensually over his genital area, and then sweep your hands up on to his abdomen.*

the flowing fan strokes which you apply to the whole upper area of her body. In the same way, massage her legs, gliding your strokes up over her inner thighs and sensitively around her groin. Take care not to intrude abruptly on to her genital area, but sweep your hand tenderly over her vulva and pubic mound.

When the woman is massaging the man, spread the oil over his skin to warm his whole body before paying special attention to his buttocks and thighs, first with soft, smooth motions then with firmer pressure. While he lays on his back, relax his abdomen with soft circular strokes, leaning closely into him so that your hair or breasts brush lightly against his skin. Gently massage over his genital area, caressing his penis and scrotum, but do not over-stimulate him. Guide his attention to other parts of his body by stroking down on to his legs or up over his chest.

A LOVING FACE MASSAGE

To touch and massage the face of your lover is a very personal act and your hands will need the awareness and sensitivity that all tantric loving requires. Your hands should be soft but steady as they move deftly over the features of the face. Your strokes will remove tension, refreshing and

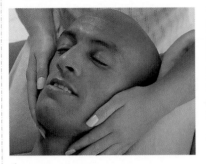

1 *Apply a small quantity of oil on to your hands. Stroke them gently, one after the other, first up over the neck, and then across the chin and jaw.*

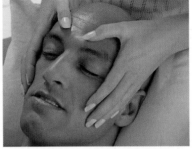

2 *Glide your thumbs steadily from the centre of the brow towards the sides of the head. Repeat the stroke up over the entire forehead.*

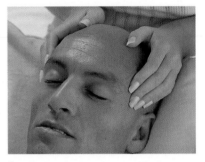

3 *Softly cup and relax your hands, circling your fingertips several times in soothing clockwise motions over your lover's temples.*

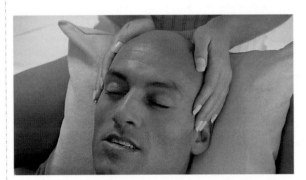

7 *Relax your hands to sweep the palms soothingly up over the sides of the temples and scalp, then draw them away from the head.*

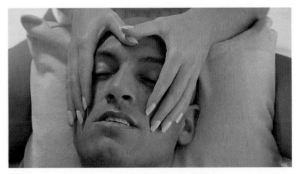

8 *Rotate your fingertips anti-clockwise on one place at a time all over the fleshy area of the cheeks and around the mouth and jaw.*

revitalizing your lover as they sweep over his or her temples, brow and jaw. A face massage will help your beloved to relax into a more spontaneous mood. It is an excellent way to start or finish a whole-body massage, or it can be enjoyed as a caring experience in its own right.

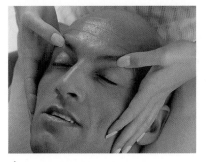

4 *Draw your thumbs from the inner to the outer edges of the eyebrows, then press the pads sensitively up into and along the brow bone.*

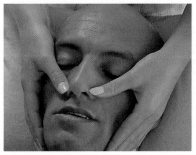

5 *Place your thumb pads each side of the bridge of the nose, then glide them firmly down to the nostrils and out towards the cheekbones.*

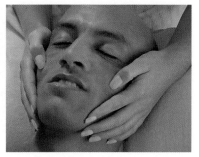

6 *Continuing from the previous stroke, slide both thumb pads directly under the cheekbones, softening the pressure at the sides of the face.*

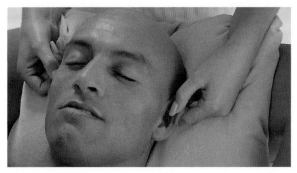

9 *Supporting the back of the ears with your index fingers, make continuous tiny circular strokes over the lobes and rims with your thumbs.*

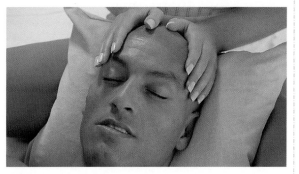

10 *Complete your face massage with a peaceful hold, cradling the head between your hands as your thumbs rest on the centre of the brow.*

A RELAXING RITUAL

Bathing and massaging your lover's feet can become one of your special rituals, serving not only to relax and refresh your partner, but also as a gift of love and devotion.

Take a bowl which is large enough to fit both feet and fill it two-thirds full with warm water. For a luxurious touch, add up to four drops of essential oil – relaxing lavender or cooling peppermint essences are perfect choices for a foot bath. For a more sensual blend, add two drops of patchouli mixed with two drops of lavender essence. Find a comfortable position for your partner to sit in and ask him or her to soak his feet for at least 10 minutes. Taking one foot at a time, lather it with soap, gently squeezing and pressing the foot all over to release any tension. Then pat each foot dry with a soft, warm towel. Now massage one foot and then the other, ensuring your partner's legs are comfortably supported and relaxed.

▼ *Take it in turns to offer each other a relaxing foot massage, ensuring that both of you benefit from receiving its stimulating and simultaneously soothing effects.*

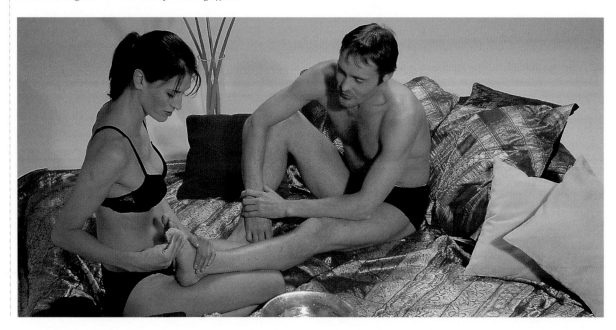

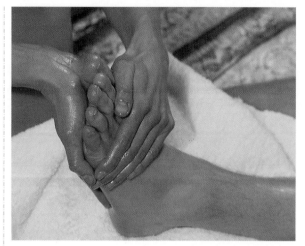

1 *Cradle each foot between your hands for up to 30 seconds to create a relaxing warmth and the feeling of caring tactile connection.*

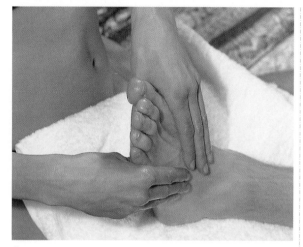

2 *Sweep your hands smoothly several times from the toes up to and around the ankle, gliding your fingers back down over the foot.*

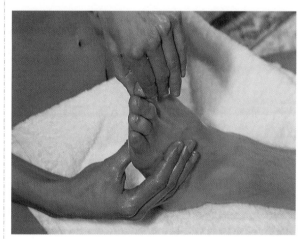

3 *Supporting the foot, stretch each toe by gripping it between your thumb and index finger and sliding firmly from the base to the tip.*

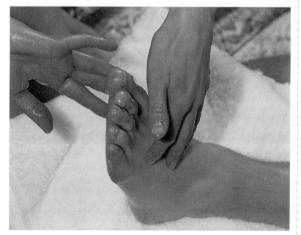

4 *Complete the foot massage with feather strokes, drawing your fingertips in soft motions down over the foot and towards the toes.*

FINDING TRANQUILLITY

The tranquillity of meditation opens the door to tantric loving. The potential of meditation is the attainment of inner equilibrium, the focus of mind and spiritual wholeness. These serene qualities are at the very root of tantric sexuality, which emanates from tranquillity rather than excitement, and from harmony not passion.

Set aside time to meditate, either alone or together. A meditation teacher can guide you through special breathing techniques or you can just sit quietly in the peace of your own home. Dedicate an area or, if possible, a specific room, purely for meditation and tantric love-making. Choose a quiet time and turn off the telephone, radio and television. Create a conducive atmosphere for your meditation by closing the curtains

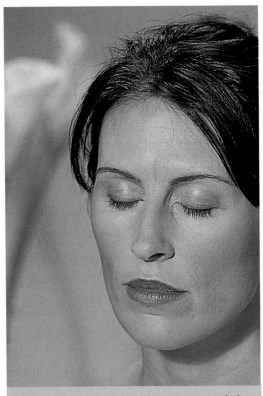

▲ *By stilling your mind and becoming one with the flow of your breath, a sense of serenity and wholeness emerges in your consciousness.*

and lighting candles, placing them on an altar converted from a low table or box. The fragrance of certain essential oils will enhance the meditative mood – you could blend three drops of cedarwood, two drops of frankincense and two drops of rose absolute to produce a spiritually uplifting and heart-opening aroma.

Sit comfortably on cushions, with your legs crossed and your spine relaxed but erect, shoulders and chest widened, and hands resting on your thighs, palms facing upwards. If you are unable to sit on the floor comfortably, sit on a chair and ensure your spine remains extended. Attention to breath is the key to meditation. Close your eyes and focus on your breath as it flows steadily in and out of your nostrils. After a while, allow your breathing to deepen, and become conscious of the rise and fall of your abdomen with each inhalation and exhalation. Whenever your attention wanders back to your thoughts, return to the awareness of your breath. The more frequently you meditate, the more you will experience precious moments of tranquillity and stillness inside yourself. Initially, you may prefer to meditate for short sessions of no more than 15 minutes, but later you can extend the sessions to 40 minutes or longer. A muffled alarm clock can alert you to when the meditation period is over. Take time to relax for some minutes before resuming your normal activities.

▼ *Sit and meditate together in a tranquil atmosphere as a regular practice. This ritual will create greater serenity within your relationship.*

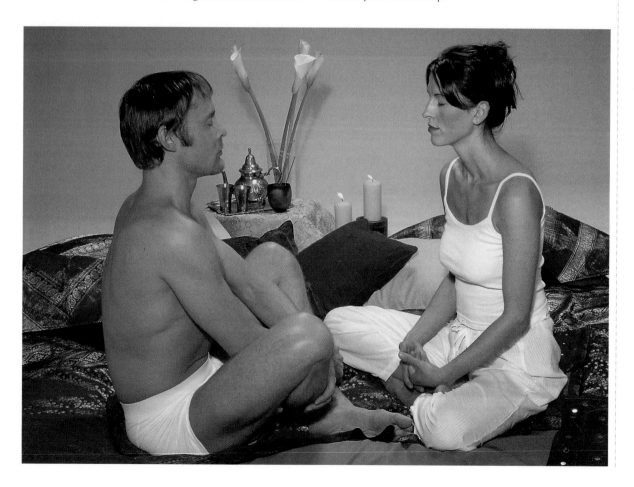

AWAKENING ENERGY

The more you meditate and the more meditative your love-making becomes, the greater the awakening of energy is within you. You may experience this awakening as a stream of vibrations, similar to an electrical current pulsating within you. If the flow of energy within you is blocked, your vitality is diminished. If your energy is streaming unimpeded, you are more in balance within yourself and with the external environment. The healthy functioning of the chakras, or energy centres, also affects your normal psychological, emotional and physical health. You are more able to fulfil your potential in matters of survival, sexuality, power, love, communication, intellect, intuition and spirituality.

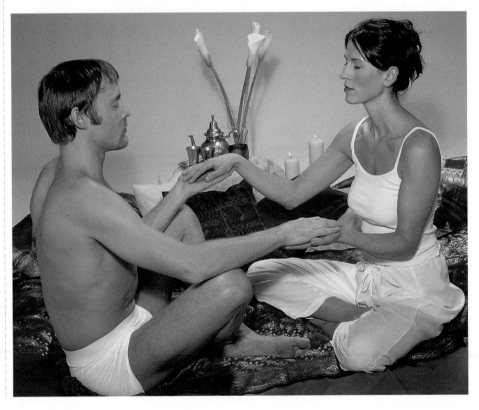

◀ *Start by creating a circuit of energy between you for five minutes. Place your right palm over your beloved's left palm. Imagine that you are receiving energy as you inhale, and sharing it as you exhale.*

Meditate upon the chakras by directing awareness and breath to their specific locations within your body, and by becoming more sensitive to their subtle vibrations and associated feelings. Go back to the "Chakra Chart" in the Introduction and familiarize yourself with the location and qualities of each chakra. Sit quietly in a meditative posture and focus your breath and awareness on each chakra for approximately three minutes at a time, beginning with the base chakra and moving gradually up towards the crown. Visualize the luminous rainbow colour related to each chakra as your breath connects with it. Complete the meditation by sweeping back down the central channel in your body with your breath until you return to the base chakra. Always take time to rest after a chakra meditation.

A potent chakra meditation is to sit body to body in close contact, breathing into each chakra for three minutes as before, beginning with the base chakra and moving up towards the crown, while visualizing that your energy centres are unfolding like the petals of a flower.

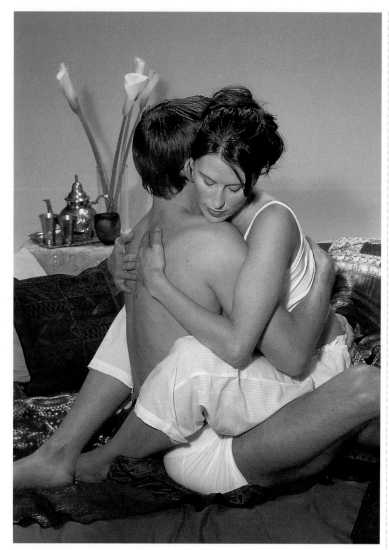

▲ *Merging your bodies close together, synchronize your breathing as you focus for three minutes on each chakra. Complete by sweeping your breath back down from the crown to the base chakra.*

MERGING SEXUAL ENERGY

When you unite sexually on an energetic level, so that movement arises spontaneously and without effort, love-making can feel almost bodiless, as if you are dancing and merging together without the barrier of physical form. This sense of merging is at the heart of tantric loving because it harmonizes your opposing male and female energies, creating the balance and equilibrium from which ecstasy arises.

One of the most important tools of tantric love-making is deep and conscious breathing. Breath is the link between body, mind and spirit, and it ignites the body's vital energy. Breathing is an involuntary action, but when you allow it to become full and conscious your whole being is more relaxed, your body is more sensitive and you are more emotionally open. Your sexual energies will start to dissolve together when you are receptive and responsive to one another in this way.

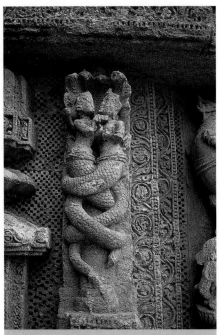

▲ *This ancient Hindu sculpture depicts the ascent of the cosmic Kundalini energy as the divine god and goddess merge in sexual ecstacy.*

Tantric loving involves intimacy, connection, stillness and merging. As such, it is very different from normal sexual behaviour, which is very active and sometimes almost aggressive, involving a lot of "doing", stimulation and arousal. Fantasies are often the driving force behind normal sexual excitement, but they can create a distance between you, almost as if you were making love to a different person. If you are obsessed with the idea that orgasm is the only proof of good sex, then your sexual performance may become fraught with anxiety and effort.

Cultivate stillness in your sexual relationship, allowing movement to arise spontaneously rather than by design. Take time during love-making to stop and merge with each other by lying entwined in each other's arms, breathing deeply together with soft-focus eye contact and savouring every tiny sensation that vibrates through you. Whenever you feel you are losing the intimacy that bonds you together, slow down so that you can again fall into harmony.

▶ *Gentle pelvic movements will keep your lover erect whilst inside of you without over-stimulating him as you lie together in deep communion.*

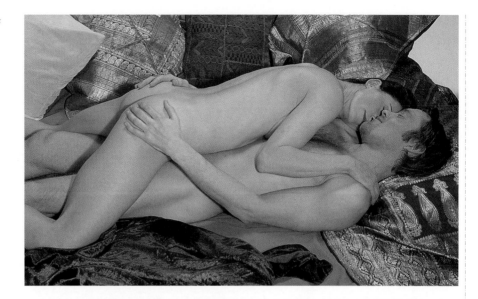

▶ *Moments of stillness in your love-making create a space for intimacy to deepen. Through your breathing and your eye contact, you will become more harmonious.*

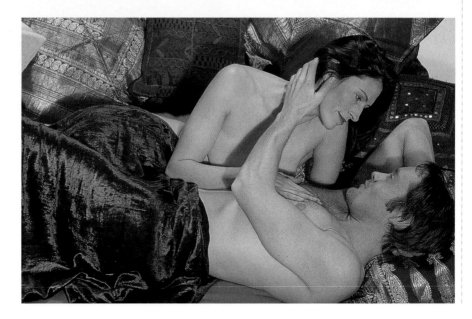

ONENESS WITH NATURE

Experiencing oneness with Existence is the basic tenet of Tantra. It teaches that we, like every manifest aspect of Nature, are part of Cosmic Creation, which arises from the perfect and harmonious union of male and female universal energies. In lovemaking, meditation and our relationship with the external natural environment, we can taste the bliss that arises from such communion.

Submerge yourselves in the natural wonder of Existence by making a serious commitment to break away from both domestic and work responsibilities on a regular basis to rediscover together the magic of creation. Go to a beach on a warm moonlit night; lie and gaze at the stars and listen to the roar of the ocean or the gentle lapping of the waves. Walk through a forest and explore the myriad life systems that exist within it, or stroll across a soft carpet of meadow grass and search for wild flowers. Sit by a river and listen to the bird song, watching the insects dance and buzz above the water. Together celebrate the power of creation, feeling yourselves to be part of its splendour.

Become attuned to the five elements of Existence (earth, water, fire, air and space), which, says tantric law, are each related to one of the first five chakras of the body. According to Eastern tradition, all aspects of life contain the five elements, and harmony and health are created when they co-exist in balance with one another. Tantra teaches that ecstatic love-making brings equilibrium to the five elements within our bodies, renewing our vitality and

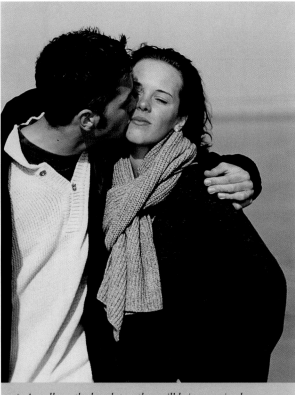

▲ *A walk on the beach together will bring you in close contact with the elements of Nature.*

happiness. When you are out in the natural world with your beloved, be conscious of the elements. Walk barefoot to touch the earth beneath you; bathe in water to refresh both body and mind; let the warmth of the sun kiss your face; allow the breeze to brush your skin and gaze into the emptiness of the sky to see infinity. Carry home with you an awareness of the divine nature of Existence, and as you make love acknowledge that you and your beloved are part of it.

▶ *The silence of meadows and forests offer a haven of peace for lovers to enjoy one another's company.*

▼ *The majestic beauty of snow-capped mountains can evoke within you a deep sense of oneness with Existence.*

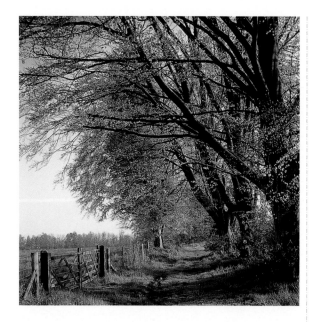

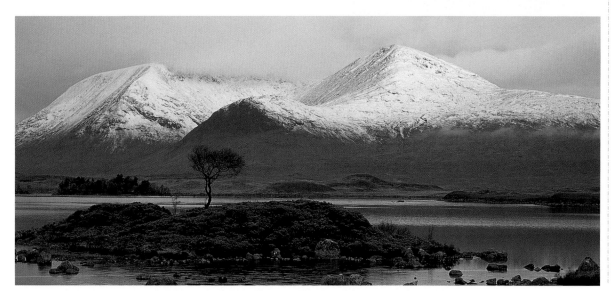

THE FIVE SENSES

Tantra teaches that the body is the temple of the spirit, and through its senses you can begin to experience the ecstatic and divine nature of Existence. Live life to the full, embracing pleasure and sensuality, but at the same time bring awareness into every action that you make.

The body's capacity for pleasure is experienced through the senses: smell, taste, sight, touch and sound. They are related, in that order, to the first five chakras: the base, navel, solar plexus, heart and throat. By involving your senses fully in your interaction with the world around you, and in your love-making, you increase your capacity for joy. Do not allow your senses to become dulled. Create specific occasions, with or without your partner, when you stimulate one particular sense at a time so that your appreciation of the joys of life, and of each other, becomes more acute.

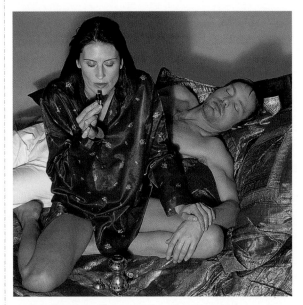

▲ *Delight in special fragrances and explore the evocative effects on your moods from inhaling the abundant natural aromas that surround you.*

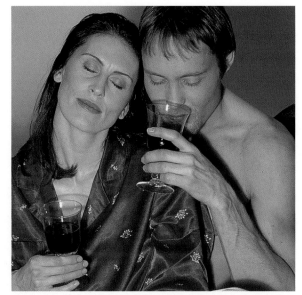

▲ *Appreciate your food and drink, eating and sipping slowly to savour each individual flavour, so that eating and drinking become a true celebration.*

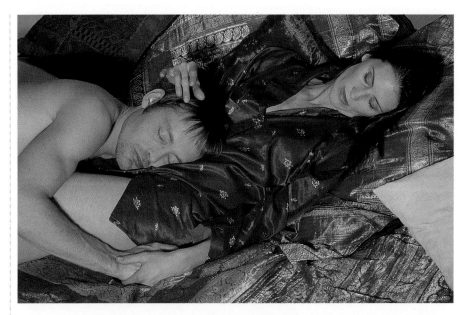

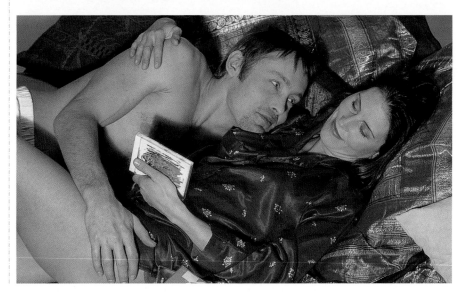

Allow your hands to become sensitive and responsive when touching. Let them convey your feelings whenever you caress your lover.

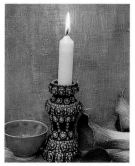

Gaze into the flickering flame of a candle in a darkened room, softly focusing on the light. Relax your eyes so that you absorb rather than stare at objects.

Lay quietly with your partner and listen to music. Increase your appreciation for the gift of sound, listening attentively to the song of a bird and the sounds of Nature.

A SANCTUARY OF LOVE

The environment where you choose to make love should be considered with great care so that its ambience is both sensually and spiritually uplifting. When you go into this area with your beloved, you should feel as if you are entering a sanctuary of love, dedicated to the enhancement of your tantric union.

Tantric disciples in ancient India took great care to select or create a hallowed atmosphere in which to partake in sexual rituals, believing that the external environment exercised a strong influence on the state of body, mind and spirit. Colour, materials, aromas, flowers, objects, sound and lighting were believed to stimulate the senses and activate the chakras, so that the tantric lovers became more receptive to each other and to the divine nature of their sexual union.

▼ *The right choice of materials, perfumes, candles and flowers can create an uplifting love-making environment.*

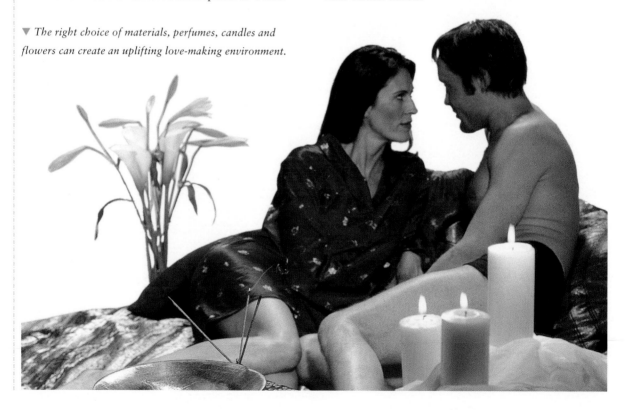

Create your love nest tenderly and with care so that its atmosphere supports and heightens the whole experience of your love-making. Remove any clutter and unsightly objects from the room and from under the bed. Cover the bed with soft natural fabrics in colours that are warm, earthy, romantic and pleasing to your eye. Or drape soft material around the bed to create an inner sanctum. Tantric colours are traditionally ochre, red and orange, which are said to stimulate sexuality. Fill the space with soft pillows and large cushions on which you can relax, or use to support your bodies comfortably.

Light candles to bathe your skin in their gentle glow, and perfume the air with essential oils in an aroma burner, using a blend of aphrodisiac and spiritually uplifting scents. Place beautiful flowers on an altar dedicated to your love for each other. Add objects that are romantically meaningful to you both alongside them. Music may help to inspire your mood, relaxing and opening you up to each other.

Try to keep this tenderly created space exclusively for your meditation and love-making rituals.

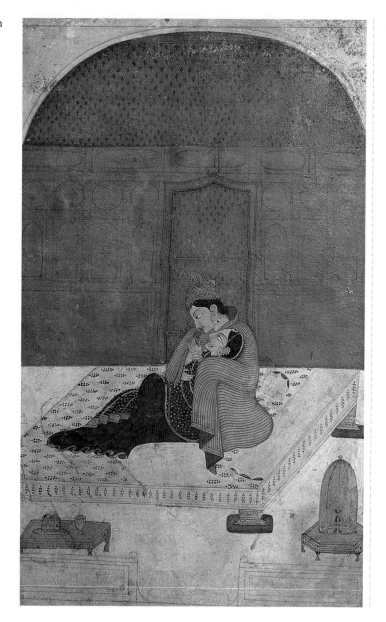

▶ *This Indian artwork from c. 1800 depicts a love chamber which was especially prepared for the romancing couple.*

DIVINE LOVE-MAKING

Commit yourselves to your love-making, ensuring that it is central to your lives as a couple. Even when you feel overloaded with other responsibilities, make a conscious choice to nurture your sexual relationship. Consider it to be of primary importance to your physical, emotional and spiritual development together. Tantric love-making is an invitation for the sacred to enter into your sexual union. It is a ritualized act, inspired by the consciousness that you are evoking the essential divinity within yourself and within your lover.

Organize your times for tantric love-making carefully, so that you do not feel that you have to rush. Prepare your tantric space so it is warm, perfumed, aesthetic and welcoming. Bathe and anoint your bodies so they

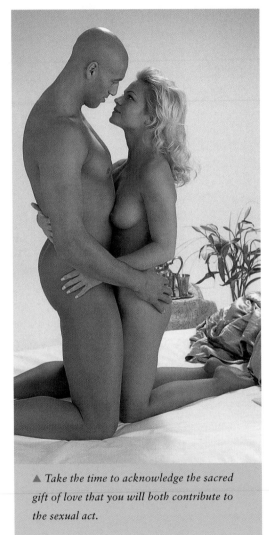

▲ *Take the time to acknowledge the sacred gift of love that you will both contribute to the sexual act.*

feel fresh, purified and sensually enlivened. Sit within your room and meditate together to acquire a sense of inner peace and harmony with each other. Enjoy a small meal of delicious snacks and fruits, beautifully arranged on a tray, and feed each other titbits to stimulate your tastebuds. Offer each other a glass of wine or fresh fruit juice to sip from to celebrate the occasion. If you desire, you can massage each other, perhaps a foot or a face massage, or one of you can offer a whole-body massage to the other.

Lie still and entwined with each other, harmonizing your breathing and allowing your bodies to melt together. Kiss and stroke each other so that your caresses touch over the whole body to gently awaken the sexual energy.

Perceive in each other the image of a god and goddess so that every touch is one of reverence. Honour one another's bodies as the gateway to the divine, bestowing kisses on the most intimate areas as if in an act of worship. Relax into the warm surge of sexual arousal, breathing deeply into your pelvic area and letting the sensations course up through your entire body away from the genital areas. Visualize your sexual energy moving up through each chakra with each exhalation of breath. Return to stillness whenever one of you becomes over-excited and release all thoughts of a goal to this love-making session. Orgasm may or may not happen, but it is no longer the purpose of your sexual encounter. Instead, you are meeting and merging in an act of deep and divine communion.

▼ *Tantric love-making is a joyous exploration of your physical and spiritual nature.*

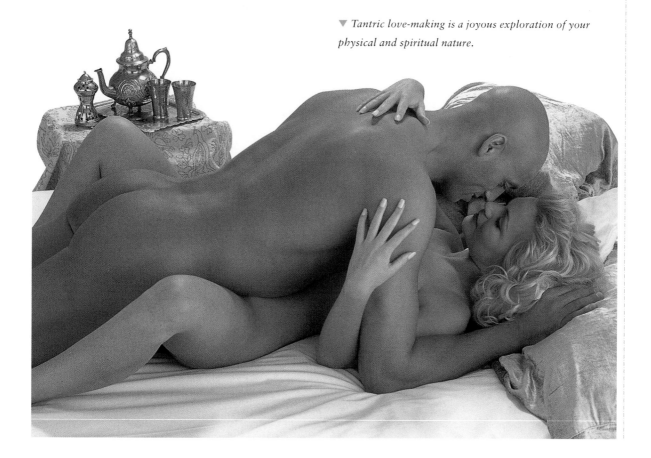

THE MAN'S CONSCIOUS PASSION

As the male, you must learn to moderate your sexual excitement so that you can retain control of your arousal levels and thus avoid ejaculation, at least until a moment that is mutually satisfying for yourself and your partner. You must make love to your lover selflessly, ensuring that she reaches the full potential of her sexual satisfaction. Avoid losing yourself in fantasy or rushing headlong into a whirlpool of excitement. Instead try to remain in the moment, intimately connected to your partner. Focus on your lover as the goddess of your dreams, so that your caresses adore every part of her body. Relax into this "plateau" level of arousal, consciously staying below the threshold of orgasm and dissolving into a deep state of relaxed sensuality.

▲ *When your passion overheats, stop thrusting and become still.*
Lifting your head, steady your breath and focus your thoughts.

▶ *Regain your control and equilibrium whenever you become over-excited. Hold each other closely and breathe deeply together.*

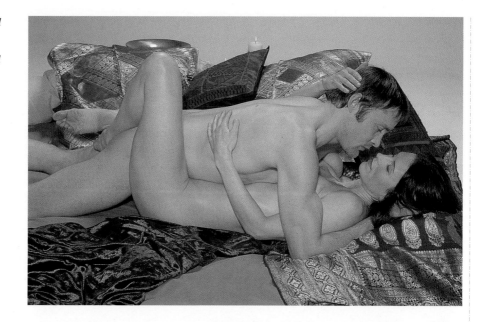

▶ *Try and explore different positions that help you retain control. When your lover raises her legs on to your shoulders, you are able to penetrate deeply without becoming over-stimulated.*

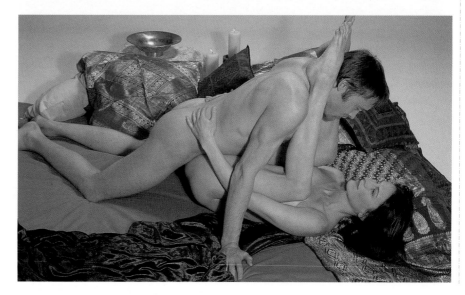

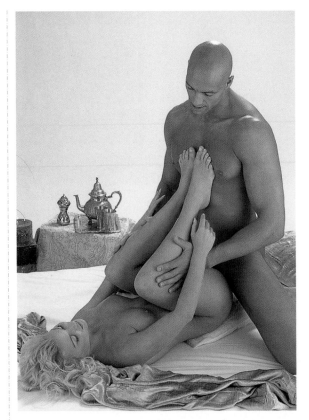

▲ *With her body compact and her feet pressed against your heart chakra, she can surrender herself to your strength and masculine presence.*

Cool your passion by slowing down movement, closing your eyes, inhaling steadily through your nostrils and focusing your thoughts on your breath or some other fixed point. Avoid panting as this will lead to loss of control. Be aware of your patterns of thrusting, and if over-aroused withdraw your penis to

rest at the opening of your lover's vagina until you regain your equilibrium. Hold each other tightly and breathe together. Tantra teaches that the woman's vaginal juices give strength to the man, so as you relax together in this position imagine that you are absorbing her secretions into yourself. Resume deep thrusting only when you have gained control over your arousal level.

The advanced yogic techniques of traditional tantric disciples require years of dedicated discipline and guidance from an accomplished teacher. However, a few of the semen-retention techniques can be adapted into your love-making. Like many Eastern traditions, Tantra is aware of the energy body and the pathway of its meridians. It suggests applying pressure on certain meridian points to steady the mind, cool the passions and avoid early ejaculation. If you feel close to ejaculation, arch your spine, lift your head upwards and breathe deeply, at the same time applying pressure with the index and middle finger of your left hand on to the area between your scrotum and anus, thus inhibiting the flow of semen from the prostate gland. Another technique is to press your tongue against the roof of your mouth while steadying your thought and breath, or to roll up your tongue and use it like a straw to draw in cooling air.

Feel confident in your masculinity and strength, for to your lover you should become like a god to her goddess. Yet also allow the soft, sensual and more sensitive aspect of your sexual nature to emerge, so that the more feminine side of yourself integrates

with your maleness. Learn to surrender yourself
to your lover's orgasmic nature, allowing her the
freedom to express herself, and dedicate yourself
to her happiness.

Experiment with different love-making positions
that bring pleasure to you both but that enable you,

▼ *The "spoons" position of love-making is perfect for times
of stillness and merging during sexual union. Gentle
movements of the pelvis will ensure the man remains erect.*

as the man, to stay in greater control of your orgasm.
Do not over-emphasize these techniques, otherwise
your love-making will become wooden and
unspontaneous. The ability to stay naturally in the
"plateau" phase of love-making becomes easier the
more it is practised. Your body and mind will adapt
to a whole new way of sexual response so that love-
making increasingly functions from a meditative and
relaxed state of being rather than from titillation,
excitement and tension.

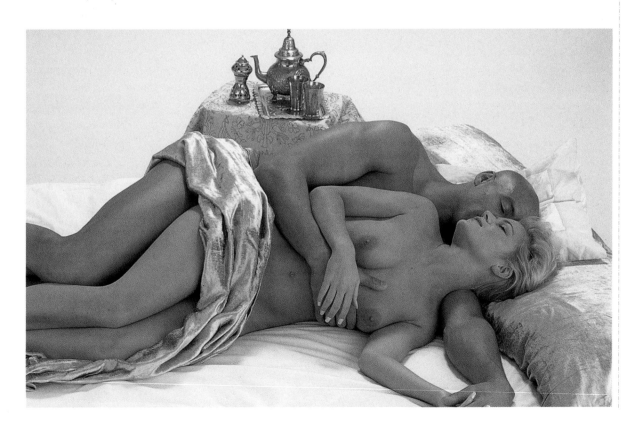

THE SEXUAL POWER OF A WOMAN

Tantric loving is very liberating and affirming to your femininity and to your sexuality as a woman. In tantric tradition, the woman is perceived as the creative instigator of sexual energy and the medium through which it is transformed into ecstasy.

Your sexual happiness and fulfilment should be of utmost importance. Your body is to be revered for, according to Tantra, it is the divine instrument of sacred sex. No part of your body can be considered embarrassing or shameful, for in Tantra your vulva and vagina are the heavenly gates to the journey of bliss, and your secretions are the nectar that brings harmony and balance between yourself and your lover. Your orgasmic nature is celebrated in tantric loving, for it is recognized that a woman is likely to gain in energy as she climaxes. Tantra allows you to be as orgasmic as you wish so long as you stay aware and connected with your

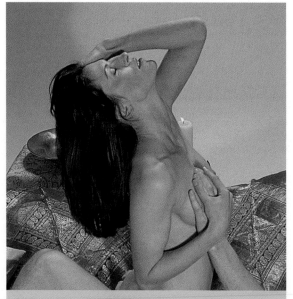

▲ *Be wild, untamed and ecstatic but remain conscious of his arousal level.*

lover, assisting him to prolong his love-making. Do not be afraid to assert yourself sexually, adopting the superior position. Sit astride him while he submits to you and lies inert on his back. Take charge of the depth of penetration and the movements so that he can focus on his breath and inner stillness.

Channel your orgasmic energy upwards to vibrate through your whole body. Relax and breathe deeply into the sensations, moving your body and emitting the sounds and sighs that arise naturally in you. Visualize your sexual energy ascending through every chakra, each one unfolding like the petals of a flower. Fall into moments of stillness and silence with your lover, holding him close and cherishing him. Surrender yourself to him, and honour his sexual organs, touching and kissing his genitals as if in an act of worship. Acknowledge him as the divine male principle within your love-making.

▶ *Clasping his thighs between yours, tighten and pulsate your vaginal muscles to help maintain his erection while you attune deeply to one other.*

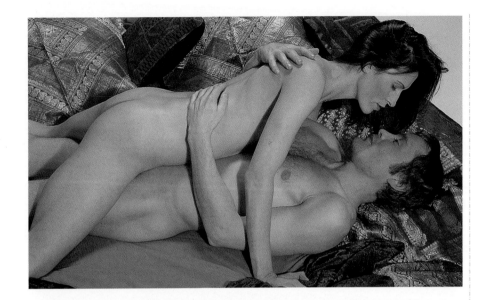

▶ *If you are supple enough, arch your whole body backwards and breathe deeply to open up the chakras to the rising orgasmic energy.*

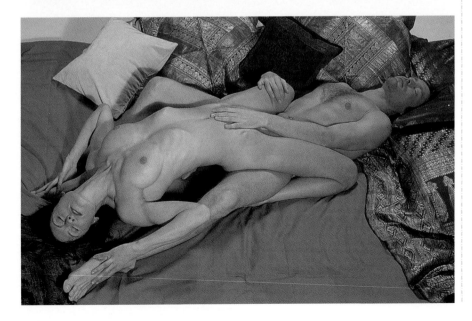

ECSTATIC LOVE-MAKING

The key to ecstatic love-making is in the sense of merging, whereby you feel as if the two of you are one body, one soul and one flowing stream of energy. You are in such a deep state of union that there appears to be no distinction between your male and female entities. It is as if your female lover has integrated into you, the man, and your male lover has dissolved into you, the woman. By becoming so attuned to one another, you will begin to experience within your own body the sensations that your partner is feeling. This means that not only are you making love to your external lover, but in doing so you are able to connect to your own inner male or female aspect, so that you can become whole within yourself.

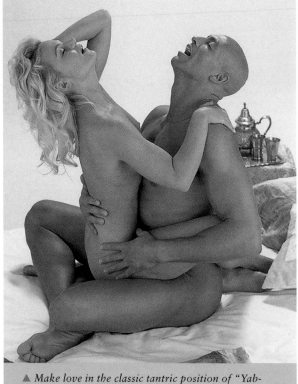

▲ *Make love in the classic tantric position of "Yab-Yum", where the woman sits on her partner's lap, and gently moves her pelvis as she enters into the state of sexual ecstasy.*

Consequently, your own bi-polar energies are unified.

In tantric love-making, your aim is to absorb your orgasmic energy into yourself so that it ascends towards the crown chakra, which is traditionally the seat of tantric bliss. Even if the concept of energy, chakras and altered consciousness is not meaningful to you, the stillness and meditation that you have introduced into your love-making will itself create a sense of harmony and joy that both of you will be able to experience.

Certain sexual positions are favoured by Tantra to create ecstatic and meditative love-making. When you both assume a sitting position and your spines are erect, the pose helps the man to moderate his passion. Your postures are equally balanced and neither of you is taking the dominant or submissive role. Energy can flow easily upwards through the spine and you are attuned to each other chakra by chakra. Breathing together, swaying gently and melting body to body, allow a feeling of benediction to descend on you. Remember, there is no goal to achieve in your love-making except to touch the sacred in one another. Orgasm may or may not happen, but if you have allowed its vibrant energy to transport you to another realm of sexual consciousness and now wish to surrender to its powerful pulsations, let go together into its blissful release.

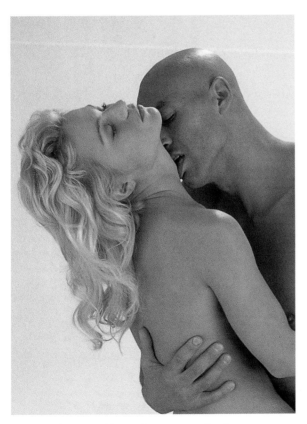

▲ *Surrender yourself entirely to one another in your love-making so that you become one body, one soul and one flowing movement of joyous energy.*

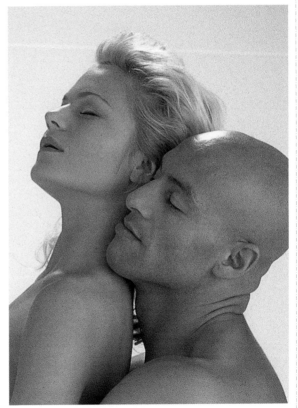

▲ *After love-making, rest peacefully together so that you remain intimately connected while you return slowly to your own sense of self.*

INDEX

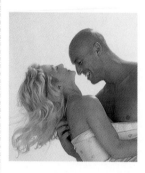
Picture Credits

The publishers would like to thank the following for supplying photographs:

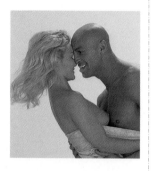

Dinodia Picture Agency, Bombay p.6 (*m*), p.10 (*br*), p.46;
Tony Stone Images p.48, p.49 (*tr*) and (*b*);
e.t. archive p. 24, p. 53;
Mary Evans Picture Library p.8 (*l*);
Ancient Art and Architecture Collection p.9 (*t*).

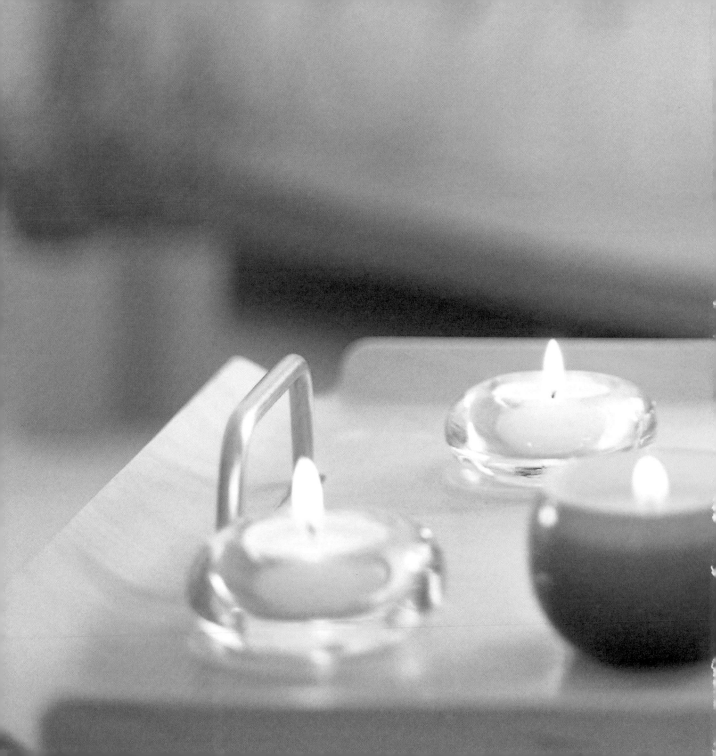